Miracles of

The Medicinal Heali

Prevention, Healii

By

Suzanne Sanders

Published by:

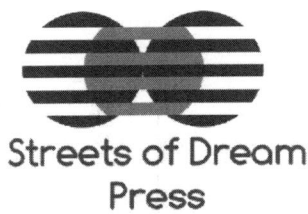

Streets of Dream
Press

Streets of Dream Press

Cover & Interior designed

By

Laurie Lanier

First Edition

TABLE OF CONTENTS

Disclaimer:

The content of this book is for informational purposes only. Nothing in this book is intended to replace diagnosis by or consultation with your personal professional health-care provider. Furthermore, no statements in this book has been reviewed by the U.S. Food and Drug Administration. Do not add any dietary supplements to your regime until you consult with your physician.

INTRODUCTION

The Chaga mushroom.

The mushroom of immortality. A gift from God. A diamond of the forest.

It's one of the most exciting natural foods in the public's eye today. While you may not have heard about it, that doesn't mean it's a Johnny-come-lately untested fad.

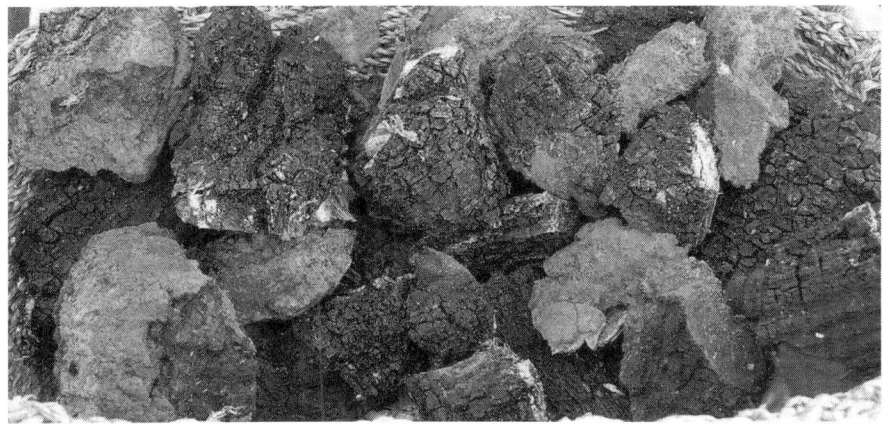

It's been used in the cold-climate regions of the world for centuries, even thousands of years.

It seems to have any number of health-giving characteristics with more being discovered all the time.

If you've never heard of this remarkable fungus, you're in for a pleasant surprise. If you're facing poor health or a particular health issue and no one has ever directed you to this natural food, then you'll be amazed, to say the least. My guess is you'll feel hopeful at first, then excited, and after all is said and done, empowered and in control of your own life.

How do I know this?

Because it's exactly the journey, I took investigating this powerful gift from Mother Nature.

You see, a good friend introduced me to the amazing health-giving powers of this one-of-kind fungus when my health had hit rock bottom. I was diagnosed with the same type of cancer my mother died of when she was only 56. I received my diagnosis when I was fifty-five and a half years-old – almost to the day.

I froze for a moment at what I may be facing. *What if I only had six months to live?*

Oh, no. I quickly chased that thought from my mind, locked it out, and refused even to pay attention when it asked to step in again. As soon as I did that, I turned to the doctor who diagnosed me and said I "wasn't going anywhere." I had a daughter I needed more time with, and a novel to finish writing (my first, by the way).

I need to tell you right now, I did not abandon modern conventional treatment, but I tailored other "treatments" to suit my needs and my beliefs, and the Chaga mushroom was high on the list.

I meditated and visualized. But frankly, until I discovered the chaga mushroom, it didn't seem like my health improved much.

Of course, I was skeptical of all the natural health powers it allegedly possessed. Of course, I didn't run out to buy chaga immediately.

And even when my research was completed, I *still* hesitated trying it. I'm not sure what the exact moment was that tipped me into putting it into my newfound health routine.

All I know is, I did, and I haven't looked back or regretted a single minute of it. And now, after surpassing my mom's lifespan by seven years, I owe it to everyone facing any type of health problem today to spread the good news about chaga.

So many people were impressed about my attitude toward cancer and the treatments. Well-meaning individuals came up to me, thinking I wasn't aware of it, stating that chemotherapy destroys not only your body's "bad" bacteria but also wipes out all of your "good" or healthy, necessary bacteria.

When I told them I was well aware of that, they looked at me amazed. Then they said in the next breath that chemotherapy also weakened my immune system. I again repeated I knew that.

But I'm a firm believer that if I have some legitimate treatment within my reach, then I need to indeed reach for it and give it an honest try. So, I added it into my diet along with my meditation and visualization routine.

At first glance, you'll be skeptical. Most individuals are, even when they're told of the diverse health benefits from regulating glucose levels and lowering cholesterol, to helping control and maybe even prevent cancer.

That's only natural.

That's why this book covers in as much detail as possible (some of it a bit scientifically) why even scientific researchers and the conventional medical community are watching and studying the results of every new research paper that studies the chaga.

SEVEN YEARS AND COUNTING

That was seven years ago. Yes, you read that right. For the last seven years, I've been drinking several cups of chaga tea on any given day and making delicious desserts that included chaga in various forms. I chastise friends who say the cancer is in remission; I'm cancer-free, and it isn't returning. Period. No need to talk about it any further.

My story isn't unique. There are more people than you know using chaga mushroom as a tea or in meals and now, thanks to its current popularity, in any number of forms as supplements.

In the seven and more years I've been using it, the mushroom's availability has skyrocketed. If you decide after reading this publication that you may like to give it a try, your search for the form of the supplement will be easy.

WHAT YOU'LL FIND IN THIS BOOK

We'll describe the fungus for you and why it doesn't look like your ordinary mushroom that may be sprinkled about your yard at the end of heavy rainfall. Not only that, but you'll want to read the unusual way most of the Western World heard about this amazing mushroom, as it's not the usual way good news spreads about a healing herb like this one.

We'll show you how it works and what diseases and disorders it's the most effective on. As you go through your investigation wondering if chaga is right for you, we'll also provide you with some recipes which help you improve your health and keep it running smoothly for years to come.

CHAPTER 1: CHAGA: WHAT IS IT?

When I was a child, I was lucky enough to have a grandmother who would let me walk around her huge yard after a good rain.

I said "lucky enough" because my grandmother, who came over from Eastern Europe and never went to high school, let alone college, taught me some of the best biology lessons I've ever received.

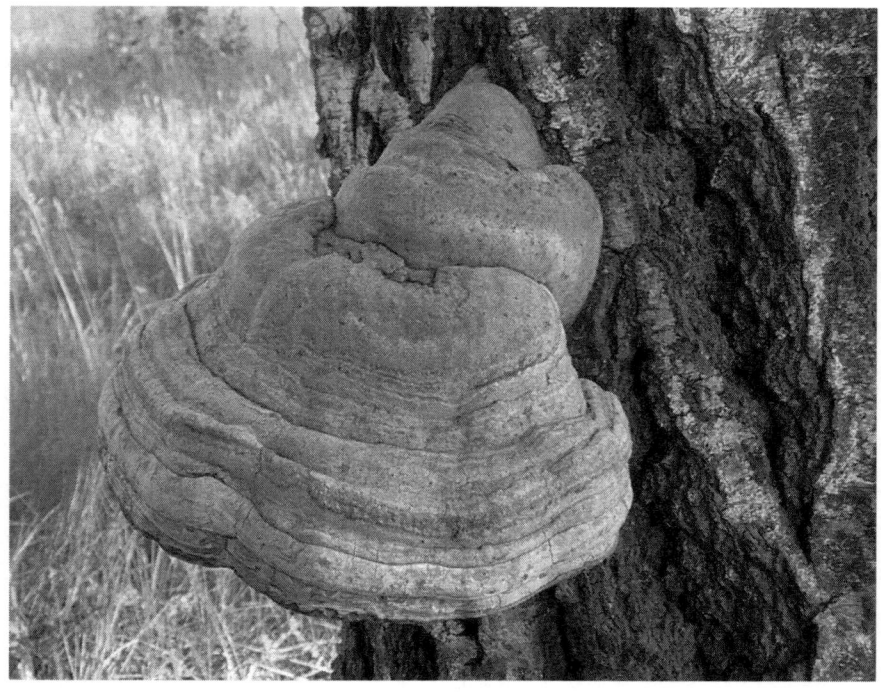

(Credit: Wikipedia.org)

I watched for the longest time, her head lowered, her eyes never leaving the ground. Occasionally, she'd bend over, pick up something, studied it, and then decided whether to stash it in her apron.

Some of whatever she was looking for would go straight to the pockets of her full-body apron, others she tossed aside.

When her pockets were full, she would begin carrying these things by bringing her apron up and creating a large basket of sorts.

One day, I rushed out of my house to see for myself what she could possibly be doing. She was searching for mushrooms that were safe to eat. That's when I got my first lesson in selecting mushrooms.

But we never found a chaga mushroom, with good reason: Chaga doesn't pop up from the ground after a good rainfall, like nearly every other mushroom. No, if you want a good look at this fungus in its natural state, you'd be wise to walk into the woods and check out the bark on trees.

EVER SEE A THIRTY-POUND MUSHROOM?

Then you've never seen chaga in its native space. Chaga mushrooms as large as 30 pounds have been found on the bark of birch trees. How big is this?

Well, some individuals swear when they find the large examples, they're the size of a human head. And unlike the more familiar forms of mushrooms, you can also find the fungus in any number of shapes up to 12 inches in diameter.

In this way, chaga resembles moss more than mushrooms. But it is, indeed, a fungus. If you're serious about finding it, you'd have to look on the birch trees of Alaska, northern Canada, and Siberia. All cold climates.

In fact, the first several times you go hunting for it, you may pass over the mushroom entirely. If you don't look closely, you may simply dismiss chaga as burnt wood.

This unique growth has sparked a discussion among many botanists on whether chaga should even be classified as a mushroom. Another difference between "true" mushrooms is its exterior. This fungus possesses a hard exterior has been compared to burnt charcoal. It's also rust-colored on the inside.

The chaga is not injuring the trees nor the result of an injury. Rather, the mushrooms and trees actually enjoy a symbiotic relationship. That means, as you'll recall from your high school biology class, that they aid in each other's healthy growth. Not only that, the chaga can help birch trees stay healthy. There has been more than one instance in which chaga has helped nurse a tree suffering from any number of diseases back to health.

In addition, the chaga mushroom needs to be soaked in hot water even a short time before it releases its amazing healing properties. The water encourages the breakdown of the tough, hard cellular walls.

TRADITIONAL USES OF CHAGA

Researchers are now finding out that some of the same chemicals, phytonutrients, and other substances that heal "sick" birches have been used to help people heal from any number of health disorders.

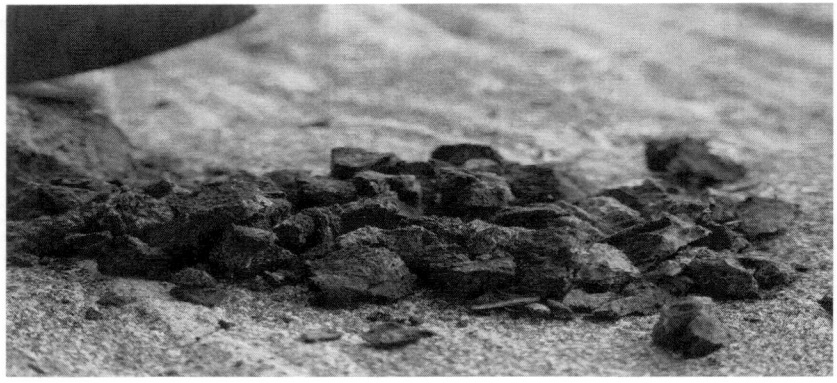

For literally thousands of years, people have been using this mushroom for an array of health disorders. Consider this; native Siberians don't hesitate to grind it into a powder and add it to stews and soups. They say it gives them something they desperately need in the cold climate: an increase in their endurance.

The bottom line is that Siberians, with their shockingly cold weather conditions, used this fungus as a standard part of the average person's diet. Perhaps that's, why for the longest time, the mushroom received little to no attention as a medicinal medium. The majority of individuals who drank it saw it as a warm tea or coffee or a culinary herb for other foods.

What the researchers either didn't know or didn't bother to research for the longest time, was the incredibly low rate of cancer and other degenerative diseases among those who added the chaga mushroom into their diet.

As early as the 11th century the indigenous people of Siberia, the Khanty, used this mushroom for more than just nourishment in their food. They had already discovered that when they drank the chaga as a tea, it helped to calm their digestion.

They smoked the fungus with the aim, so it's said, to prevent lung cancer. And yes, that certainly seems counterintuitive. They converted it into soap to help heal skin sores.

Not only that, but the Russian people recognized the healing power of this mushroom, along with a few other cold weather mushrooms.

As far back as the 12th century, that would be the 1100s, traditionally-trained and highly respected healers were reportedly successful in treating Tsar Vladimir Monomakh's cancerous lip tumor with chaga.

While for the most part, the Siberians' use was quite normal, eventually the word spread by visitors to the area who were amazed at the quality of health and seeming absence of disease.

Soon, the stories of the amazing powers of this unique fungus made its way to the Baltic Sea and other areas, where the Chinese and Japanese quickly discovered its therapeutic values. This led to the indigenous people of Ainu in Hokkaido who drank it with the specific goal of improving their overall health as well as boosting their immune system.

Aside from those benefits, it also appears to protect from the development of many degenerative diseases that are far too common in the United States. Epidemiologists, scientists who study the demographics of populations, note that Siberians have greater life spans than many populations who don't use chaga.

One of the most amazing aspects of this cold-climate population is their low rate of cancer compared to others around the world.

Siberians, though, aren't the only people who have a long tradition of including the chaga mushroom as part of an overall healing treatment for various disorders. Many of those growing up in Eastern European countries have used it as a treatment for a variety of skin conditions, including eczema and many respiratory disorders, including bronchitis.

Traditional Chinese medicine practitioners as well as Korean healers also put chaga to good use – and have for thousands of years. And of course, even today, it's been used regularly.

HISTORY OF TREATMENT: FROM STOMACH PROBLEMS TO SKIN DISORDERS

But that's only the tip of the iceberg when it comes to a history of chaga's medicinal potency. The first verifiable known use of this mushroom come to us from 16th-century Russian texts. These books explain that it was regularly used as a treatment for what we call today gastric ulcers and gastritis.

The doctors of that age would encourage their patients to make a tea from it and slowly sip on it all day long. It was effective in reducing intestinal pain as well as quelling upset stomachs.

BOOST YOUR ENERGY

Historically, the mushroom has also been known for its ability to alleviate hunger and increase energy. It was a go-to ingredient in teas and soups for cold-climate hunters and forestry workers.

In addition to calming the stomach, chaga has a reputation for successfully treating skin conditions. It has a long, successful history of reducing or eliminating the symptoms of eczema and psoriasis.

Finally, in testimony to its effectiveness on maintaining healthy skin, the Khanty people of Siberia burnt the mushroom and added it to hot water. They called this "soap water" and used it as a disinfectant, a substance that kills bacteria.

Fast forward to World War I and World War II where this superfood was used to make a coffee substitute

Now that researchers are turning their attention to the verification of these wives' tales, they've come across with surprisingly good results. This seems ironic since many people have found chaga on trees often dismissed as a cancerous tumor on the tree itself.

In the next chapter, I show you only a small slice of the exciting news the super-powers this mushroom appears to have.

CHAPTER 2: HEALTH BENEFITS

Until I began investigating the health benefits of the chaga mushroom for my own healing, I wasn't aware of how it can improve health, whether you're dealing with a serious illness or just giving your system an energy and nutritional boost.

Trust me; when I first began my own research, I was more than a bit skeptical, not only about the wonderful health-giving characteristics of this fungus but also when it came to considering any adverse effects.

First, I tackled the research that would verify the benefits. If I could discover and confirm these, then I would check out any adverse effects. Then and only then would I place the pros next to the cons and make a logical decision.

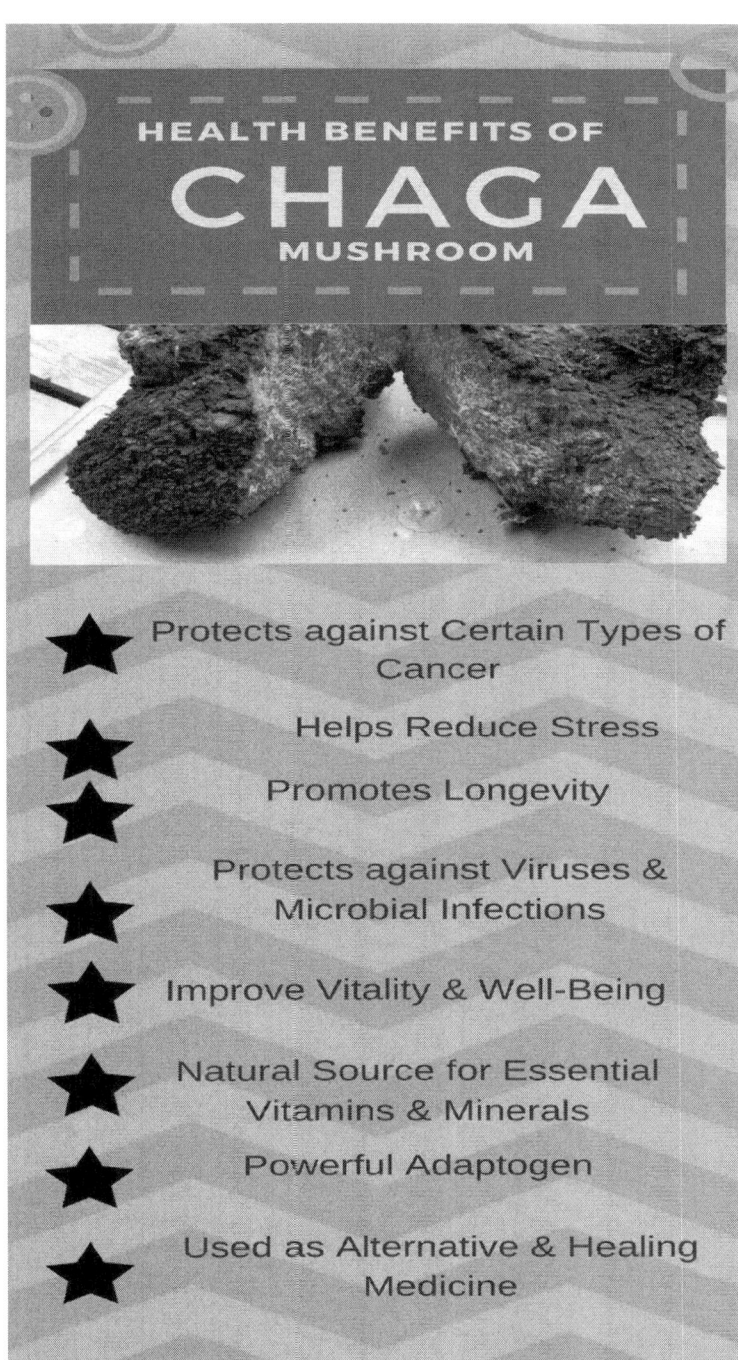

HEALTH BENEFITS OF

CHAGA

MUSHROOM

- Protects against Certain Types of Cancer
- Helps Reduce Stress
- Promotes Longevity
- Protects against Viruses & Microbial Infections
- Improve Vitality & Well-Being
- Natural Source for Essential Vitamins & Minerals
- Powerful Adaptogen
- Used as Alternative & Healing Medicine

TOO GOOD TO BE TRUE?

I've always lived by the motto: If it sounds too good to be true, it probably is. So, as my research found that the benefits of this herbal supplement mounted, so did my skepticism. But there was still a voice in my mind that argued, what if it isn't too good to be true?

JAM-PACKED WITH ANTIOXIDANTS

First, the chaga mushroom is rich in antioxidants. These are substances found in a variety of the healthiest foods that help to keep the development of degenerative diseases at bay. In addition to that, chaga is low in fat, sugar, carbohydrates, and even calories.

BOOSTS YOUR IMMUNE SYSTEM

Again, research involving humans is scarce; the studies involving animals are quite successful. Chaga mushroom appears to possess substances that can kick start a sagging immune system. Why is this important? When your immune system isn't producing enough white cells, it isn't providing your body with

enough protection from the common cold and the
Not only that, low immune systems may make it
harder for you to manage everyday stress and make
you more susceptible to it injuring your health.

The medical community believes that one of the ways
in which this mushroom works its wonders is because
it stimulates the production of spleen lymphocytes,
which are necessary for healthy and strong immune
systems.

REDUCES INFLAMMATION

This amazing fungus reduces inflammation, according
to preliminary research performed with animals. One
study revealed that the extract of this mushroom
reduces inflammation triggered by ulcerative colitis.

INCREASES STAMINA

It's true. Animal studies found that those that took
chaga extract experienced greater physical stamina. A
study published in 2015 discovered that mice given
chaga polysaccharides exercised, in this instance
swam, longer than those who didn't take the

substance. Not only that, but the fuel – glycogen – content of both muscles and liver increased while lactic acid levels in the blood decreased.

ANTI-VIRAL PROPERTIES

In addition to that, there's more data coming out almost daily that chaga extract contains potent anti-viral properties. One of the most recent studies revealed that the mushroom has this effect on your body's immunodeficiency virus or HIV.

Experiments performed with animals confirmed, at least tentatively, that this characteristic is especially effective on hepatitis C virus. What occurred, in a nutshell, is the anti-infection properties of the virus plummeted by a whopping 100-fold, and it only took 10 minutes. Of course, research on the anti-viral abilities of chaga continues, but based on this small start, the results should make the community take a second and third look at this amazing mushroom.

What does that mean for the future of the mushroom? You'll find that chaga is an excellent candidate as an ingredient in future antiviral drug development for

many of our most stubborn diseases and disorders.
The future never looked better.

CHAPTER 3: CHAGA AND HEALTH DISORDERS

If the list of this mushroom's health-giving benefits is impressive, then actually applying them to some of the toughest diseases and disorders facing us in the 21st century is an exciting adventure in healing.

Translating these factors into the potential healing powers for a wide range of stubborn diseases, diseases that are tough to heal, diseases in which many cases have no known cures, and diseases that are far more likely to develop as people go through the aging process gave me a wake-up call.

It was at this point that my skepticism melted slowly. As I read some of the research on the various disorders chaga allegedly could heal, I could begin to look at the picture of its gifts.

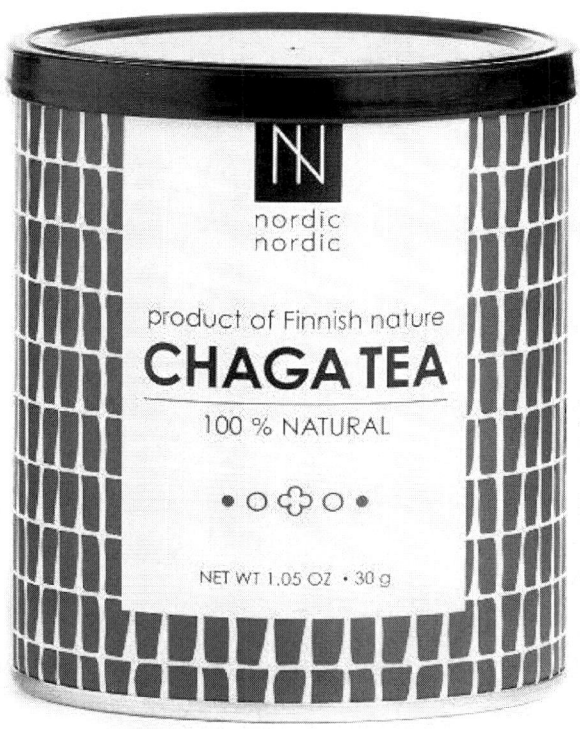

CHAGA AND CANCER

It's a curious route that turned chaga into a known alternative to cancer treatment.

Up until the 1970s, the mushroom was practically unknown. You might think someone brought some of the fungus back from a vacation or from a visit to a relative. That would seem justifiable. But no, that's not how the majority of Americans learned of it, even if they didn't realize what was happening at the time.

Believe it or not, Americans can thank the bestselling Russian author Alexander Solzhenitsyn who wrote The Cancer Ward.

In this book, he gave us a stunning look of what this fungus can do for cancer patients.
Skeptical, but nonetheless intrigued, medical researchers had to check out the mushroom for themselves. While they probably thought the words of Solzhenitsyn were embellished to enhance the plot, researchers felt they had a medical obligation to study this fungus in more depth.

They felt they had nothing to lose, and the potential for an effective cancer treatment center to gain. Inaction, indifference, and skepticism were inevitably overridden not only by intense academic curiosity but also by an obligation to the many people who had or may develop cancer.

So, what did the researchers discover?

The found out the area in question talked in broad brushstrokes about cancer, but the bottom line proved most amazing and worthy of further serious research. None of the several residents in this area were reported entering the hospital because of cancer. Not a one, they were told. In almost the same breath, they were also told that the vast majority of the parents in this region would save money on their coffee by cutting back on the grounds and mixing them in with the powdered mushroom instead.

When they went out into the nearby forests to investigate this fungus, they were startled to discover one thing. The total number of pathogens, or substances that can kill bacteria and viruses, was far less found in one operating room in a modern hospital.

This means that, in plain language, you'd have a stronger chance of picking up a cold, virus, or other diseases by standing in that operating room than by standing in the forest. Why?

The mushroom uses those same pathogens in its symbiotic relationship with its host tree, successfully using its antibacterial properties to ward off invading pathogens and keeping the host healthy.

How does Chaga do this?

Normally, I shy away from explanations that involve too much chemistry and analysis of the substances of plants or disorders. But the news the chaga brings to the world of cancer is so exciting, that I can't help but talk about it. Don't worry; I'll make it as simple to understand without distorting the process.

One of the reasons I'm doing this is because so many individuals become very skeptical when you mention any alternative cancer treatments, which is why they really need to check out what this fungus can do. The first substance I'm going to introduce you to is polysaccharides and beta glucans. These two substances of the Chaga fungus are its two main active ingredients. They give Chaga the ability to boost your energy levels as well as your brain and liver functions.

Betulin, also known as betulinic acid, is the substance that has the ability to kill cancer cells without injuring, damaging, or even stopping the growth of the healthy cells of the body. For anyone who has been through the ordeal of chemotherapy, it sounds like a miracle.

While it does indeed sound miraculous, there is a warning that can't be emphasized enough. If you are undergoing chemotherapy at the moment, do not halt it if you decide to use Chaga as a tea or in any form at all. You may want to bring up the topic with your oncologist to ensure that the combination doesn't produce adverse effects. Certainly, don't take it upon yourself to disrupt this medical treatment.

The medical community is finally taking notice of the potential healing powers of chaga on cancer. "Laboratory and animal studies show that chaga can inhibit cancer progression."

That statement was made by the well-respected Memorial Sloan Cancer Center and is potentially explosive regarding the future of cancer treatment. The institute urges that more studies using individuals with cancer need to be conducted. There have been several experiments conducted on mice, which proved to be quite impressive, as well as hopeful.

One study observed mice who had cancerous tumors and supplemented their diets with chaga. Remarkably, 60 percent of the mice experienced a reduction in the size of the tumors. What's more, the mice also experienced a 25 percent drop in tumors that had spread to other areas of their bodies compared to the control group.

In a separate scientific study published in the professional journal, **World Journal of Gastroenterology,** the effects of the mushroom on cancerous liver cells of humans was analyzed.

The results? The research revealed that chaga extract appears to have the ability to prevent liver cancer cell growth. More investigations need to be performed, but it certainly is good news that chaga may be used as an alternative treatment for liver cancer

Another way that chaga may protect you from the risk of cancer development is its power to attack coagulated blood. This mushroom thins your blood which is one of the many reasons why it's also beneficial to your heart.

But what you may not know is that cancer cells thrive in an environment that contains thicker blood. Obviously, the opposite is also true. Thinner blood that is blood that has difficulty coagulating puts you at less risk of developing cancer.

HALTING MICROBE GROWTH

Microbes are the bacteria that actually cause disease. Because of the high concentration of phytosterols in this mushroom, as well as lanosterol and inotodiol (also known as phytochemicals and phenols), microbe growth is halted and controlled.

Chaga contains the highest antioxidant count of all medicinal mushrooms.

That's right. Antioxidants are legendary not only in preventing cancer, but rather treating it as well. That's because this fungus contains the active chemical substance of melanin. We'll talk more about this substance, as well as melatonin, after covering ut the mushroom's ability to aid in the function of your pineal gland.

There's still one more factor you can't ignore when you're talking about the high antioxidant content of chaga. This humble fungus also has more capabilities in this area than mega servings or vitamins C, A, E, co-enzyme Q10, spirulina, and grape seed extract, and beta-Carotene.

But you don't have to take my word for it. A study, conducted by the University of Mississippi, was published in the *American Chemical Society and American Society of Pharmacognosy* journal several years ago. It revealed that the chemical substances we've just talked about are what gives chaga its "strong anti-microbial" properties.

Chaga is a great source of new antibiotics. In other words, the study concluded that it has "shown direct anticancer effects." Additionally, the research concluded this tree fungus also has the capability of actually preventing the metastasis, or spread of cancer to other parts of the body.

But how do I use it?

While I would never recommend that you use the alternative medication in place of conventional cancer treatment, it at the very least can be used as an effective insurance policy before you're diagnosed. This is especially true if you have a family history of cancer.

HEART DISEASE, YOUR CARDIOVASCULAR SYSTEM, AND CHAGA

It's been said throughout the centuries that mushrooms – a wide variety of them – are known to be "food for the heart." In recent years, scientific studies have confirmed the age-old wisdom of our ancestors. Studies have shown that those who eat mushrooms or use mushroom extract, including chaga, are at a smaller risk of heart disease than those who don't eat the fungi, drink their tea variations, or use supplements in some form.

So, it should come as no surprise that chaga is vital to robust heart health and an unimpeded cardiovascular system. Part of the reason for this amazing contrast, medical studies show, is the presence of heart-healthy minerals known as selenium and manganese.

There's more to these facts than these two minerals. A scientific study conducted by Japanese scientists and published in the reputable **Life Sciences,** a professional medical journal, confirmed this. The experiment is technical in its nature, but the results revealed something astonishing: Chaga worked because even a small bit of the fungus can give your heart an immense boost.

If that weren't enough, chaga also has an amazing effect on coagulation of the blood. As it addresses as it addresses the platelet function of your blood, preventing the excessive aggregation of blood cells, which many times if left untreated, can lead to blood clots.

Many people, having been diagnosed with heart disease or warned about their high cholesterol numbers are, at first, baffled because frankly, they feel good. Your body gives you few, if any, symptoms that your cholesterol is anything but ideal. That's why chaga is such an effective treatment regarding heart disease.

We've talked about the powerful antioxidants found in the fungus. It's this antioxidant content that makes it a potent, natural treatment for heart disease specifically by lowering cholesterol levels.

You already are far too aware of the facts of heart disease, especially if you or someone you love has been diagnosed with it. It's the largest "killer" of all diseases of adults in the United States. The truth of the matter is, one out of every three deaths in this country is due to not only heart to disease in general but also strokes.

To put this in perspective, it amounts to approximately 2,200 deaths per day. And do you know what the very first symptom of heart disease is? It's either a heart attack or a stroke. That doesn't give many people the opportunity to do much in the way of prevention of the condition.

Including chaga in your diet can change all that. Instead of living in fear that you'll receive your first "symptom" of this potentially deadly disease, you can find yourself being relieved knowing you're taking positive action for your heart and health.

If you already have a diagnosis of heart disease, or if you have a history of heart problems in your family, you may want to start drinking chaga tea. In this instance, waiting to include this fungus in your diet after you've noticed symptoms may be too little, too late.

One of the greatest aspects of this detoxifying plant is that the medical community is now beginning to think that, among all its other capabilities, it may be a vasodilator. This is a remarkable substance that has been known to open blood vessels wider, while at the same time lowering blood pressure.

The latest research on the effects of this plant on cardiovascular disease takes these explanations and goes one step further. According to some medical experts, chaga, as well as the bark of some birch trees, are actually raw kinds of cholesterol. That's right. These raw molecules are critical, therefore, for heart health.

This is an important safeguard to your arteries, considering the constant pressure your cardiovascular system is under.

Your body takes the sterols in the chaga and then incorporates them into the actual walls of the arteries and heart muscle. Why should you care? Because when your heart and arteries incorporate these raw materials, it then makes the fibers of the heart muscle more flexible.

The lack of flexibility is one of the hallmarks of heart disease. The ability to restore it means you're also improving the pumping capacity of your heart and, in turn, protecting it from injury.

For these purposes, you can simply drink the mushroom tea.

CHAGA BENEFITS THE SYMPTOMS OF ARTHRITIS

Arthritis is a joint disorder so common it really needs no introduction.
Or does it?

We all know arthritis to be the typical wear and tear of your bones after forty-some years or more of use.

And many would be quick to add that rheumatoid arthritis is its close cousin, caused when your immune system turns on its own cells, confusing them for foreign invaders and triggering an autoimmune disorder.

But what fewer individuals know is that the term 'arthritis' covers a hundred or more disorders of the joints. Some of these joint conditions you've heard of, others you haven't.

And still other joint pains you may have experienced, but never imagined they were related to arthritis. Like gout. It typically appears as an overpowering pain on one of your two big toes and is caused by an excess of uric acid. It's associated with a diet rich in beef.

I mention this because pain anywhere in your body can be explained by one simple word: inflammation. And if there's inflammation in the body, chaga can help alleviate it.

But first, just a quick lesson in the most common form of arthritis. The type you probably have or will experience at one time in your life is called osteoarthritis. It's not only characterized by pain in one or more of your joints, but also a stiffness that's worse in the mornings.

Osteoarthritis is the kind of the joint pain that most of us experience. It causes the cartilage that covers the ends of your bones at the points where they form a joint to break down.

Rheumatoid arthritis occurs through a different route. As we mentioned, it's an autoimmune disease that initially attacks the synovial lining of the joints.

Conventional medicinal treatments of these various conditions vary depending on the type and the pain level.

If you're even bothered a bit by the onset of arthritis or in pain most of the day, you're no doubt a step ahead of me. Yes, we've talked much about the seemingly miraculous anti-inflammatory potency of chaga. In fact, if you didn't know better, you'd think Mother Nature gave us chaga just to help you ease your pain and other symptoms of arthritis.

Unfortunately, few scientific studies have been performed on this mushroom and its ability to relieve arthritis. The good news, though, is that so many people have used this mushroom before you, so you can find many testimonials of people who wouldn't go a day without taking chaga in some form.

While we talked about the inflammation that triggers arthritis, medical science now has discovered much of this occurs within your stomach lining. We've talked about this with other health disorders as well.

Not only that, but some these specialists now believe that some of the inflammation may also be found in your teeth as well as your jaw bones. When the inflammation is located in these most unlikely places, they're referred to as foci of infection. The infection in these areas is the ultimate cause of the inflammation.

Few studies are being performed on this intriguing topic, but there is at last one that was performed in Korea, created specifically to study how chaga blocks inflammation. What the researchers discovered was interesting. They saw that chaga blocks production of the specific enzymes that regulate the ultimate process.

Nitric oxide synthase, which you've probably heard of, and cyclooxygenase, more widely known as COX-2, were effectively blocked by the use of this herbal remedy.

What does that mean in plain English?

These two enzymes are the most powerful mediators of inflammation known to medical science today. That decided it for the Korean researchers. Based on this data, you'd be well within the range of correctness to call chaga a "medicine." Of course, you can't refer to it as such in the United States for a variety of legal reasons, but you can begin to supplement your diet with either chaga tea or coffee knowing you're easing your pain at the source.

That's great news for those with osteoarthritis, but where does that place the person who suffers from rheumatoid arthritis, the decidedly autoimmune disease?

There's good— no, great— news for those who suffer from rheumatoid arthritis as well. The same researchers have noted that the mushroom elixir also has amazing powers to potentially activate your immune cells. In fact, the increased activation was so strong; they had no trouble measuring them.

Another study independently confirmed this. The researcher concluded that chaga had "profound effects" in its ability to not only reduce inflammation but to actually reverse it. This capability, the scientist said, could be most effective in the presence of autoimmune diseases, like rheumatoid arthritis.

According to these scientists, this makes chaga extract as potent as any of the anti-inflammatory drugs on the market today, minus the adverse side effects. If you're skeptical of these conclusions, perhaps an anecdotal piece of evidence will help.

This testimony, surprisingly, is from a medical physician, He suddenly felt pain about midway down his back. He knew it to be deep in the rib area and was so painful that he worried it might be the result of a kidney stone. When his physicians ruled this out, he was still puzzled and still suffering from the pain. He nearly screamed with every move he made. What was curious, he thought, was that it hurt even worse any time he breathed deeply.

Realizing that conventional medicine couldn't help him, he was willing to give chaga a try. At this point, he realized he had nothing to lose. So, he bought the tea and made a large cup of it. Yes, he thought the larger the cup, the better, given his level of pain.

So, he drank his first cup of chaga tea and wondered how long it would be before he could expect to feel some results. It wasn't long before he got an answer. For the first time since he acquired this unexplained pain, he actually felt it easing. He immediately went back into the kitchen and made another cup of chaga. Then another. With each cup, he felt better and better.

He then took several drops of the extract sublingually, or under the tongue. He was astonished to discover not only had the pain disappeared, but that he felt a surge of energy he hadn't experienced in years. As long as he continued taking these large servings, the pain remained at bay, and he found he was able to rise early in the morning, as he used to.

If you're currently taking prescription medication for any of your arthritic conditions, be sure to check with your personal health-care provider before using the mushroom. That being said, don't think that chaga will be able to take the place of these conventional treatments, but they are a marvelous adjunct to them.

RESPIRATORY DISORDERS AND CHAGA.

Bronchitis. Pneumonia. Even tuberculosis.

Yes. Chaga is an excellent way to alleviate symptoms of respiratory distress. You name the disorder, and it probably will be improved by regular use of chaga.

The reason it can be your best friend if you're suffering from any type of respiratory disorders – even ailments as serious as bronchitis and pneumonia – is because it acts as an antifungal agent. At the same time, this mushroom is also working in its vital roles as an immune system booster. You're already well-aware that your immune system is your first line of defense when it comes to protecting you from both bacteria, as well as viruses.

Just every health problem that deals with the lungs and breathing problems can be mitigated, many individuals insist, simply by using chaga on a regular basis. The disorders themselves are caused when various bacterial fungi get lodged into your respiratory tissues themselves and stubbornly remain there. If you don't have a strong enough immune system to pull them out of the tissues, they'll stay there and only make your symptoms worse.

That's where chaga comes in, with its immune boosting characteristics.

SINUS, PROBLEMS, AND EARACHES – AND MORE

It very well could be that you've never felt the pain and suffering of bronchitis or pneumonia. But you feel like your body is constantly under the attack of serious sinus problems or earaches.

Can chaga actually help you with these health disorders as well? Not only that, if you suffer from asthma, this amazing herbal remedy may help you with your breathing.

With regards to the herb's amazing healing power with chronic earaches, there's much anecdotal evidence backing this statement up. One of my friends experienced a stubborn, chronic earache for nearly a year. Visit after visit to her doctors and others were futile. No prescription medication helped. No treatment eased the pain. She now was to the point where a deeper, more serious health problem was at play, and this earache was only a symptom.

Of course, no doctor agreed with her, but she couldn't understand why none of the best doctors she knew couldn't find a cause. One day, she mentioned the problem to me. While I couldn't give her any guarantees, I thought she had nothing to lose if she gave chaga a chance. The worst that could happen, I told her, was that it wouldn't work.

But I was confident it would work. I had already been researching this mushroom for several years and had read about people relieved of chronic pain of all sorts. So, I told her about the fungus and how it had a great reputation for easing earaches.

Naturally, she was skeptical. But the pain was getting to be too much to bear. She decided that she would rather choose a supplement than drinking tea, so she began to take it sublingually according to the dietary supplement instructions.

She couldn't believe what happened next. She thought at first what she experienced was mere coincidence. After her first use of chaga as a sublingual supplement, she felt the pain actually lifting.

Instead of dismissing the incident, though, she continued using the chaga supplement. Today, she has been what she says is "an earache free" for nearly a year. She says with confidence that she would have no reason for the pain to return, as long as she continues taking chaga.

MENTAL HEALTH AND ALERTNESS

If you struggle with depression or other mental health issues, you may want to try this amazing mushroom. Of course, you should discuss this possibility with your personal health-care provider. Talking with him or her prior to your use of chaga, especially if you're taking medication for any mental health problems will help prevent adverse interactions with the prescription drugs you're currently taking.

Chaga possesses an abundance of a substance called sterol, which directly nourishes your brain as well as your nervous system. In effect, sterols build your system. They boost the power of your adrenal glands, for example. And, in turn, effective well-running adrenal glands are vital to keeping your brain alert and healthy.

Even if you don't have issues with mental health, chaga can work wonders on your brain. Many of us walk around in a mental fog without even realizing it until the fogginess has lifted. This fungus can kick start your mental potential. Many people who have taken chaga for any length of time report a side effect of their habit. But it's no way an adverse side effect. They have experienced an unexpected increase in their powers of mental focus as well as their ability to stay alert.

They credit chaga with giving their bodies a much-needed kick start. In other words, those individuals who took chaga for any number of reasons also discovered a decrease in mental fatigue. I'm sure you can see how this would give you the mental edge you need when, if you're a student, you're heading into final exams. But it's also a godsend when you're driving long distances or reading or writing.

This supplement, regardless of how you decide to take it, can provide your body with profound and lasting benefits and no overwhelming adverse effects.

While you certainly can drink chaga tea to get these benefits, you may want to try it as a sublingual supplement for these purposes. If you're not familiar with this class of supplements, you only need place a drop or two under your tongue. This is the quickest way to receive all of the benefits this mushroom has to offer.

We've mentioned in passing chaga's ability to help with depression. It seems to alleviate the symptoms of mild depression. It does this, according to medical specialists, through the activation of your neurons. It applies a calming effect on your body while simultaneously playing its role as an anti-anxiety agent. Partly, this occurs because of its influence on the functioning of the adrenal glands, as we've mentioned several times before.

SKIN CONDITIONS

Chaga has great benefits for your skin's health as well. You may recall from your high school science class that skin isn't just a "covering" for your body; it's the largest organ of your body, just like your heart and livers are organs of your system.

Science has a lot to say about the effects and the use of birch bark in relieving a variety of skin conditions. Chaga's effects on the skin and various skin conditions and diseases have been studied extensively.

Many of the research comes from overseas and has been so positive that it's common to find chaga as an ingredient in an assortment of skin creams from Asia to Russia and throughout Eastern Europe. It's also a go-to remedy to help fight off the symptoms of the aging process on your skin.

The creams found overseas all contain melanin, an ingredient we've already talked about with chaga. Another active ingredient in these creams is referred to by its initials, SOD, which are a collection of potent antioxidants. Additionally, the melanin works as an effective, natural sunscreen.

So, what kind of skin conditions can you expect chaga to help with? You name it, and it's probably already been used on the condition. It has proved especially powerful on chronic problems, especially eczema, rosacea, and psoriasis.

It shouldn't surprise you to learn that what all three of these disorders have in common is one trigger: the immune system.

These disorders cause problems through their ability to breakdown your tissue, which can leave an opening for infection. The disorder itself is the result of your system allowing skin bacteria and fungi in.

There are three major germs which are the culprits in this process: Pityrosporum ovale (a yeast), Staphylococcus epidermidis, and Propionibacterium acnes. It's not necessary, in reality, to know the names of these "bad guys," but you should know how they work.

One research study showed that the extract of the chaga mushroom actually inhibited the growth of these three germs. Not only that, but its sterols have the modest additional effect on the germs which specifically cause athlete's foot and toenail fungus.

If you're worried about the possible side effects because of this powerful reaction, you probably should know that in some parts of the world, this mushroom is gentle enough to help relieve diaper rash.

Earlier, we've mentioned that chaga may be a useful aid in helping ease rosacea, a relatively common skin condition, characterized by redness and visible blood vessels on your face, along with, in some instances, small bumps filled with pus.

Conventional medicine knows enough about this disorder that it's long been associated with inflammation and infection of the stomach lining. It sounds strange, but it's true. This is important to know, because you may be tempted to improve rosacea through topical means, rubbing some supplement or chaga paste on your face.

While this will help some, the best form of treatment is through tea and other internal modes. Only in this way will you get to the heart of the problem.

CHAPTER 3: CHAGA'S ADVERSE EFFECTS

The notion that natural healing aids are totally free from adverse side effects is usually erroneous. Every herb carries with it the potential of adverse effects depending on how much of the usually safe herbs you take, any prescription drugs you may be taking along with them, as well as your lifestyle.

The chaga mushroom is no different. For most people, it's not only harmless but extremely beneficial. But for some, it may mix with drugs you're taking or your physical condition.

For example, one of the more serious issues some medical professionals have with this extract is the fact it may block the absorption of specific nutrients.

Another caveat to consider if you're thinking about taking chaga is that you need to be mindful of the suggested serving size. Don't take more than that. In this particular instance, the adage 'some is good, more is better' doesn't hold. Chaga extract taken in high amounts can be toxic.

That being said, chaga normally doesn't produce side effects. But you certainly need to be able to identify them, so you know how to handle the situation.

The side effects are more common when individuals use it with prescription medication. So, before you start using chaga, be sure to check with your personal care physician so he or she can tell you what, if any, side effects you may expect.

BRUISING AND BLEEDING

Because chaga acts as an anticoagulant or makes it more difficult for your blood to clot, you may find that you bruise more easily and you may bleed a bit more.

Normally, this wouldn't be a problem, but if you're taking warfarin or low-dose aspirin to prevent clotting on top of the fungus, you may experience bruising and more bleeding than usual due to this.

Of course, the real danger is the potential that you may also be bleeding internally if you take too much. This means it would be a wise decision to take a visit to the doctor who prescribed your anticoagulant, or blood-thinning drug. He may want to lower your dosage. It normally takes almost a week for any change in drug dosage to take effect.

This ability to affect blood clotting is the reason why you should stop using the extract in any form for at least two weeks prior to any scheduled surgery. If you don't, you'll discover that you may experience excessive bleeding during and after the operation.

CHAPTER 4: CHAGA AND THE PINEAL GLAND: A GLANCE AT YOUR EMOTIONAL AND SPIRITUAL HEALTH

It's not only a little-known gland but a gland that's small in size as well. And when you ask most people if they've ever heard of it, many admit they have but are far from familiar with its purpose and its vital role in your good health.

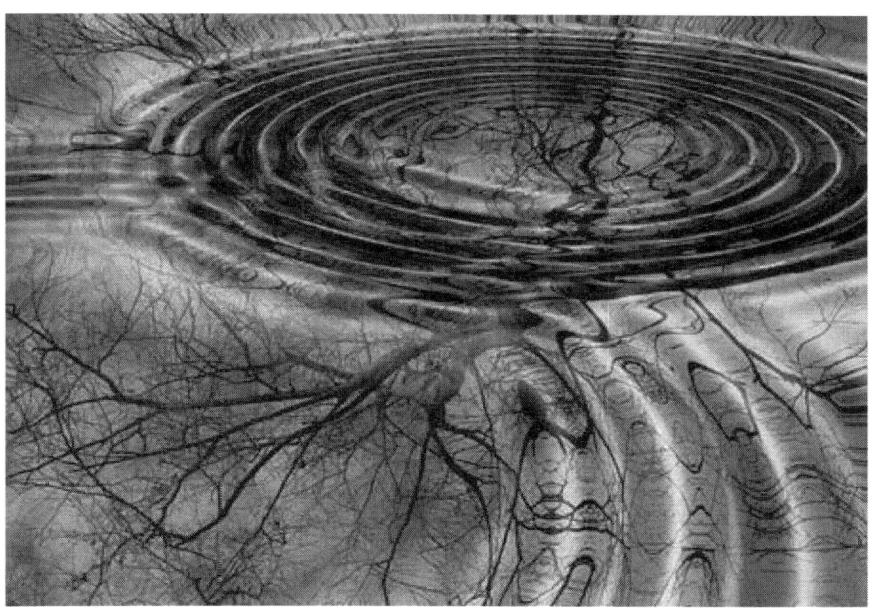

So, when you tell people that the chaga mushroom can provide the gland with a powerful boost, most individuals simply nod their heads.

Before I even talk about how chaga can increase the functioning of this gland, let's talk briefly about what a pineal gland is, how it works, and where in your body you can find it.

First, there may be a good reason why you don't hear much about this gland. When you check out the size, it's far too easy to dismiss. It's about the size of a kernel of corn. Yes, you really did read that correctly.

Where is this kernel-sized gland located? The center of your brain. Now you're beginning to get an even better picture about why few individuals know much about it.

But this small gland has a huge responsibility. It plays a vital role in the production of two specific hormones: serotonin and melatonin.

Specifically, the pineal gland converts serotonin into a form in which the gland can then release melatonin. In turn, the gland activates the gland to release another hormone known as melanocyte or MSH. This is the hormone that actually produces melanin.

Now that we have a short, but necessary biology lesson out of the way, you'll be able to see the critical importance of not only the gland but also supplementing your diet with chaga.

MELATONIN

As we look at these chemicals, we learn that melatonin is a neurotransmitter that helps maintain your sleep cycles as well as your body's biological rhythms. Not only that, but this neurotransmitter also improves your ability to sleep. Perhaps most importantly for our current discussion, is that melatonin can help boost your memory as well as regulating your moods. And if that weren't all, it also helps slow the natural aging process and contributes to strengthening your immune system.

MELANIN

Similar-sounding melanin has a set of its own responsibilities in regards to your skin pigmentation.

Melanin, created by tyrosine, is in your eyes and skin. It's your body's natural sunscreen. It also helps your system deal with daily stresses, regulates your biological rhythms, and even plays a role in protecting your body against cancer.

THE PINEAL GLAND: ALSO KNOWN AS THE THIRD EYE

So just from just a biological, secular perspective, the pineal gland is pivotal in your good health. But, this same small gland also looms large for those who are spiritually-driven, and is referred to as "the third eye." It's called this because, for thousands of years, it's been recognized as a spiritual energy source located low on your forehead, in the middle of your two physical eyes.

The third eye is a symbol of spirituality for these individuals. They assign the pineal gland this characteristic since it has the power to affect every system of your body. By extension, their logic goes at lengths to determine the potency of your intuitive awareness, as well as your consciousness.

That being said, you also need to know that, if you can improve the functioning of the pineal gland, you can boost your memories and help regulate your sleep schedule.

The gland produces one more chemical, which we're just going to call by its initials, DMT, and again, is found throughout your system. However, your pineal gland may become calcified as a result of environmental pollution and toxins in your diet.

This prevents the gland from releasing the all-important DMT, which not only helps your body but, as many argue, also helps you achieve a greater sense of spirituality and enlightenment. In turn, it hinders the release of both melatonin and melanin.

The good news is that pineal calcification can be reversed with a plant-based diet, and among those plants, chaga stands out as one of the best. Why?

The pigments found in chaga are, surprisingly, extremely similar to those pigments naturally found in your body. And with the highest concentration of melanin found anywhere in nature, the most effective way to convert melatonin is to activate your gland.

But that's not all a decalcified pineal gland capable of doing. It's effective in counteracting chronic stress and equips your body with an abundance of life-giving antioxidants, as we've already mentioned. Antioxidants specifically delay the development of cancer and heart disease, as well as other degenerative diseases.

Is there anything else you can do while drinking chaga and using it in various ways in your diet?

Yes, as a matter of fact, there is.

Spending time in direct sunlight will help hasten decalcification, as well as eating raw dark green vegetables and algae. When I say algae, I'm referencing specifically to spirulina and chlorella.

You can also improve your pineal gland function by increasing the number hours of sleep you get prior to mindset. The more water you drink, the more it will help to purify your body and cleanse your system of toxins

Some individuals also believe that exposing yourself to music and other strong vibratory frequencies will speed the improved functioning of the pineal gland. And finally, consider taking up the habit of meditation.

CHAPTER 5: HOW DO YOU GET IT AND USE IT

If you're at all familiar with herbal remedies, then you know one of the more popular ways to use medicinal plants is simply by drinking their tea, and it's no different with the chaga mushroom. Sit down to a fresh cup of chaga tea. But that's not the only choice available anymore if you've been living with this mushroom tea.

I started off using chaga tea to the exclusion of just about any other tea, and even my favorite coffee. I know this sounds strange, but there was something that just seemed "wimpy" about virtually giving up my coffee and drinking tea – even a powerful tea such as chaga.

I tried to convince myself otherwise, but I frankly missed my morning cup of coffee, strong enough that you'd swear a hand reaches out of the cup, slaps you in the face, and fully wakes you up. So you can imagine my relief and eagerness to even try a coffee and chaga mix.

And I didn't even have to worry about whether coffee would somehow detract from the mushroom's powerful health-giving benefits. Even before I took a sip of my first chaga coffee, there had already been scientific studies that analyzed the effects of this unusual drink.

One study from Finland and performed in 1958 discovered that chaga coffee was a powerful tool in the fight against breast, uterus, and liver cancers.

It took nearly a generation before more tests were performed on the coffee, which was a staple drink in some parts of Russia.

HOW TO HARVEST CHAGA

The Chaga mushroom is reaching the height of its popularity. More individuals than ever before have decided to try to use the mushroom – probably starting with small, almost "testing" steps with a cup of tea or two either once or twice a week, up to once or twice a day.

Each of these individuals have their own reason or reasons for giving a most unusual-looking mushroom a chance to boost their health.

Amazingly, more people are adding the tea to their stew or soups, finding that any level of its usage is boosting their health to a degree that they can feel it.

While that's a great natural health move in the right direction, it does cause a slight problem in other areas. It means that either these individuals are finding it more difficult to find high-quality chaga, or paying a premium price for a good extract, or both.

That leaves some people at a loss, but other more adventurous and determined individuals decide to go "mushroom hunting" themselves with the goal of finding it fresh off the birch trees.

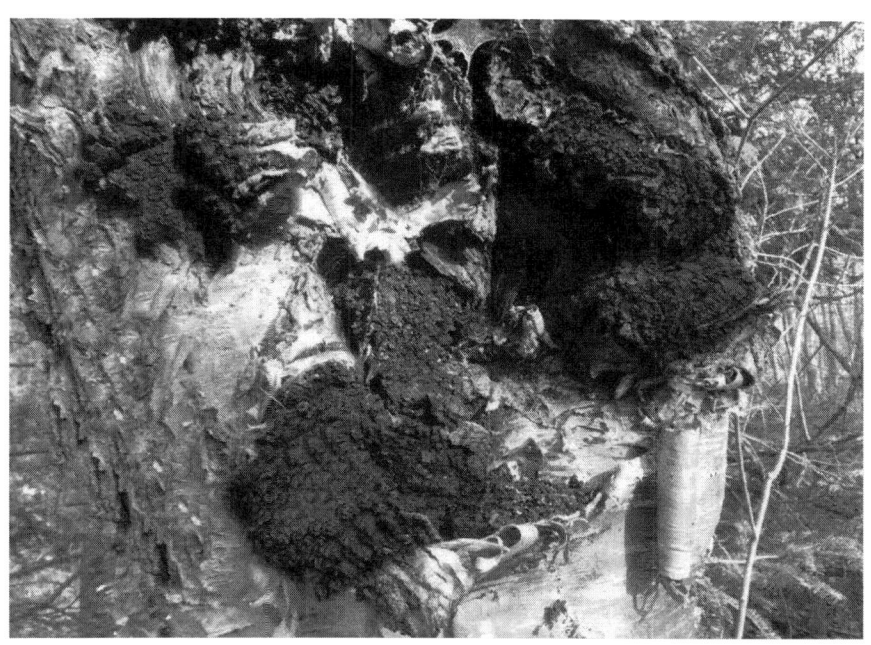

Those people living in the Northern United States and other cold areas in the country may be able to go out in search of the chaga-bearing birch trees. Once you start using chaga in this way – fresh off the tree – you may never want to go back to the prepackaged version again. Personally, I believe fresh chaga is far more effective than any packaged product you could buy.

Let me just note, this is a part of the process that I've only recently learned how to do it, but I am one of the few who actually harvests chaga on a regular basis and has studied this procedure with an eye to eventually teaching others.

My goal here is to help you, if you so decide, to harvest chaga fresh off their birch trees. Once you find the proper trees, it's really not a difficult process at all. In this way, not only are you in charge of supplementing your diet as you wish with chaga, but you're confident about having the highest and freshest mushroom you can find.

LEARN HOW TO CONFIDENTLY IDENTIFY CHAGA

First, if you decide to do this, you'll need to know what trees this fungus grows on. Chaga grows in cold regions including certain areas of the Northern Hemisphere both in the United States and Canada.

The second factor you should realize is that you should only harvest chaga from living trees. We've said that the tree and the mushroom have a symbiotic relationship. Each one keeps the other alive. Don't take a chance of gathering inert or even chaga that may ultimately be dangerous to your health.

And thirdly, don't harvest all the chaga mushrooms from the tree. Again, this is because of its symbiotic relationship to the tree. Once the tree has been stripped of its fungus, it usually dies. That's not because the chaga has poisoned the tree. Quite the contrary – the mushroom is keeping the tree healthy. Without that relationship, the host tree may, indeed, die.

I wish I could tell you that, when you're looking for this fungus, you'll be able to instantly recognize it because of its specific size and shape. But the truth of the matter is that the mushroom comes in various sizes and shapes.

Having said that, the most common forms are domes, cones, and horns with crusty ridges. The outer portion of the fungus is black, cracked, and extremely hard. It's not at all what you think a typical mushroom would resemble. If you had to compare this tough outer portion to anything, think burnt charcoal.

This outer portion is in stark contrast to the inner section which is softer and is a yellow-brown color. It almost takes on a rusty-looking appearance.

If you're planning on harvesting the fungus from birch trees, you need to know that it's found nearly exclusively on various species of birch trees in the northeast area of the continent. I've included a list of trees that are native to North America that are known to have the fungus on them.

Your search includes the paper birch tree. It's common in the northeast parts of Canada and the United States. The tree has white bark that comes off in broad, curling sheets. You can find this tree in the higher elevations of the region, as well as some of the lower ones.

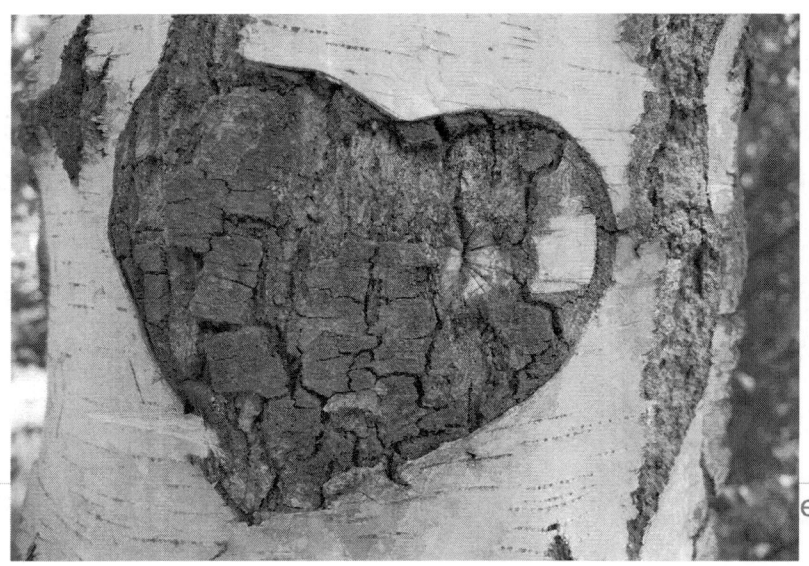
e

The yellow birch tree is also common in the forest habitat and has received its name because of its yellow bark. This bark, like that of the paper birch, comes off in small, curling shreds.

If you see a cherry birch tree, you should search for it as well. This type of birch is found in the more southern areas – relatively-speaking. Unlike its northern cousins, the bark of these trees doesn't simply pull off, and it has a deeper cherry color. The bark of this tree is smaller than that of the paper birch, and in addition to the cherry color, also contains some pink, salmon, and orange colored bark.

Don't pass up a chance to search the tree that's called the heart-leaved paper birch tree for chaga too. It's similar to the paper birch but is found mostly in higher elevations. The bark, as you might expect, looks quite like that of its cousin, the paper birch, but it also contains patches of salmon, pink, and orange-colored bark.

HARVEST TIME

Many individuals wonder if there is a certain time of the year to harvest or gather the chaga. After all, there's a specific season that you tap trees for maple syrup. And I tell them that there definitely is one for this fungus as well.

You'll get the best results if you harvest in the fall and specifically after 20 straight nights of 40 degrees Fahrenheit or lower. You need to wait because this is when the birch tree has already entered its winter dormancy period, and at the same time, the chaga is at its peak in nutritional value.

If you wait for those days, you can harvest the mushroom throughout the fall until the sap begins to run. The running of the sap signals the summer months for the tree. It's at this time that chaga will have a large water content. With a water content that can be as high as 80 percent of the fungus, it's at its lowest nutrient content. You get the picture, I'm sure.

That means you'll have to wait to collect chaga until the following autumn season. This is when the trees start collecting their water and nutrients for the following winter.

Only take chaga from living trees.

That's right. We noted this at the beginning of the book, and it's worth refreshing your memory again. The birch and chaga have a symbiotic relationship, that's true. But don't forget that, ultimately, the chaga is the parasite.

What does this mean?

For our purposes, it means that when the tree begins to die, the chaga is clinging to the tree also begins to die.

So, the next question I'm sure you're asking is, how can you tell when a birch tree begins to die?

If the tree is alive, then during its growing season you'll see the vibrant green leaves. Not every branch may have leaves, but the leaves that are there should be green. But remember, we're collecting chaga in the winter months when there are no leaves anywhere on the tree. This makes it a bit more difficult to determine its state.

If you're looking at yellow and cherry birch trees, the branches that are alive will smell like a wintergreen fragrance.

One of the things you really should be careful of doing is taking all the chaga off the tree. Whatever you do, leave some behind on the bark. This helps keep the chaga healthy, and it allows the crusty outer portion, the sclerotia of the mushroom to regrow. Many individuals suggest that you leave at least 15 to 20 percent of the fungus on the tree.

If the tree has sclerotia, leave at least one behind, and preferably untouched. This is responsible sustainable harvesting.

One more caveat about choosing the best of the fungi on the birch: if you can avoid the smaller specimens. Allow them to remain for another season. Most harvesters urge others not to take any samples smaller than the size of a grapefruit, which would be approximately seven to 10 pounds.

CHAGA AND ENVIRONMENTAL POLLUTION

Don't do yourself a disservice. If you're going through all the effort of harvesting fresh chaga, you're obviously searching for the highest quality and most effective mushrooms.

The way to ensure this is by going into areas of forest that are clean of any environmental issues. Walk far enough into the woods that you aren't bothered by any environmental pollution and other toxins. Just remember that the deeper into the forest you go, the less environmental pollution of urban areas there will be.

Wait, before you take the mushroom from that selected birch tree, you need to see the best and healthiest samples. You won't find them near the highway. To find an area like this, you need to be off the beaten path – in several ways. You shouldn't pick these mushrooms off trees that are close to a highway, for example.

REMOVING THE FUNGI FROM THE TREE

When you find chaga with a larger conk, you must extract the mushroom from the tree with care. The fungus doesn't have a stem, like an apple, where you can just snap off the stem from the tree and voila, you have a healthy apple intact.

Keep in mind as you go to remove it from the tree that you should leave up to 20 percent of the fungus on the tree for the ultimate health and life of both the fungus and the tree.

Using a high-quality large outdoor knife or axe cut the chaga from the tree without cutting into the tree itself.

Once you have the amount of Chaga you believe you'll use, that's not the end of your job. The fungus needs to be properly prepared – otherwise it'll mold and will be of no use to you. The first thing you'll need to do is dry the fungus.

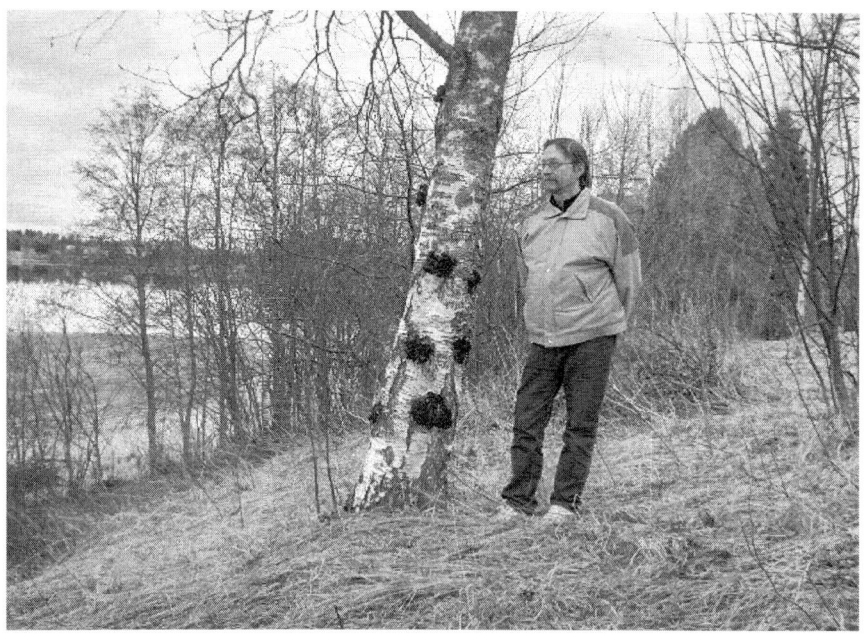

No doubt you've cut off the largest sizes you could find. During the drying process, you'll want to take these large pieces and divide them into smaller pieces that will dry quicker.

Take these chunks and put them on a pan, a sheet, or even a tarp that's near a heat source. Do not, under any circumstances, place them in the oven. You can put them near a sunny window or even a wood-burning stove if you happen to have one. Another way to dry them is to place them in a dehydrator at not more 120 degrees Fahrenheit.

In the next chapter, I've placed several recipes for chaga tea, both hot and iced. Some of the recipes, though, call for a tincture of chaga. If you're not familiar with herbal remedies, you may not know what a tincture is – let alone how you can use it.

Of course, you can always buy good quality tinctures, but for those of you who have harvested fresh mushrooms and would like to try making your own, check out the directions below. You'll be astounded at how easy it is.

To get started off on the right foot, let's look at what a tincture is. It's an alcoholic derivative of herbs, plants, and of course, mushrooms. For those of you who would rather not use alcohol as a base, or it goes against your religious beliefs, you can substitute it for distilled vinegar. The tincture will work as effectively with vinegar as with alcohol.

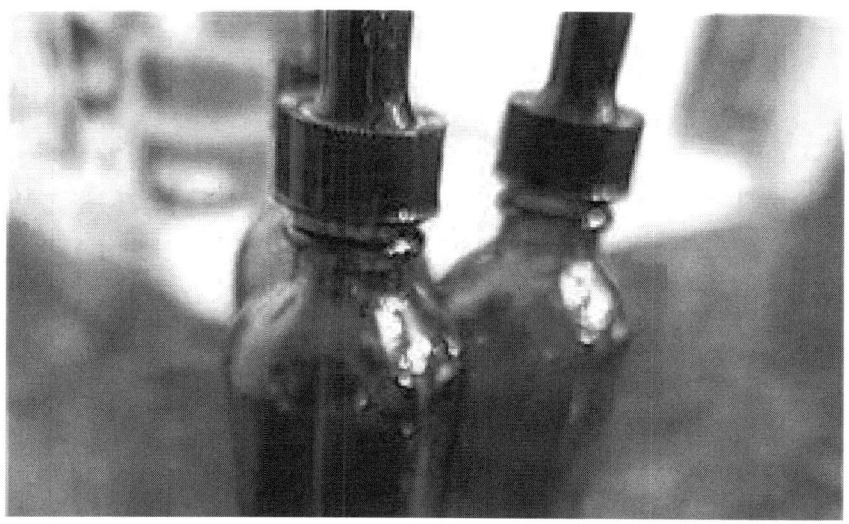

Tinctures are more effective in extracting the medicinal components of the chaga mushroom and preserving them for longer periods of time. Those who have used tinctures are pleased with how easy they are to administer, and how quickly they are absorbed by your body.

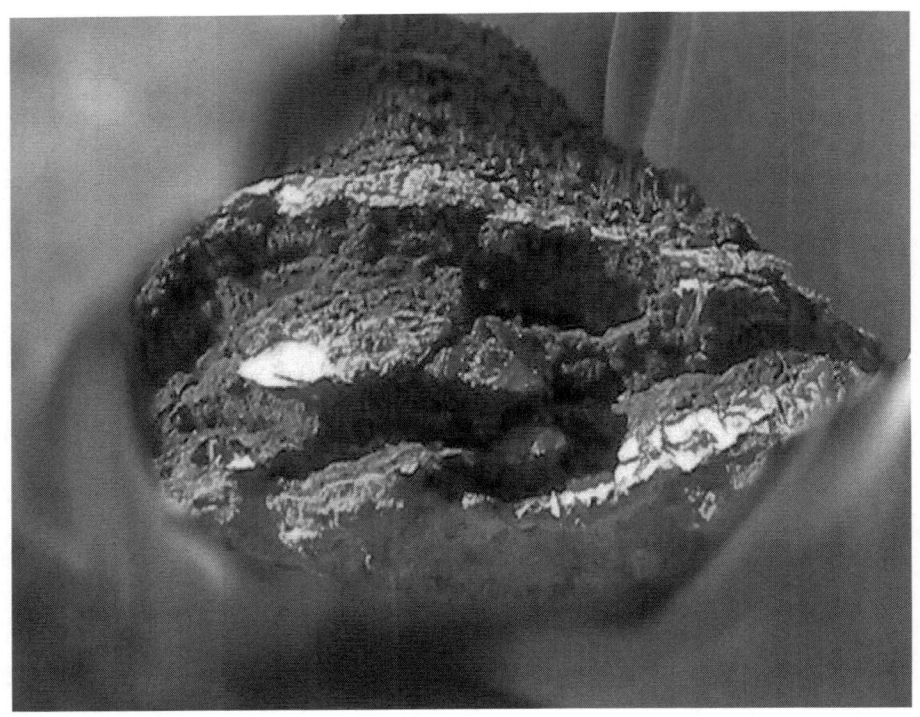

EXTRACTION METHODS

The tincture is probably the easiest way to add the healing properties of the mushroom into recipes and some drinks.

This method draws some of the most beneficial water-insoluble portions of the herb, especially betulinic acid as well as phytosterols. Hot water alone doesn't always extract these so your body can use them. Most of the time, this alcoholic extraction process is used side-by-side the hot water process to ensure many beneficial nutrients and phytosterols are drawn out.

INGREDIENTS

Chaga chunks, ground into powder to nearly fill a one-gallon jar.
Alcohol, 80 percent proof. I use vodka, but you can use whatever kind you'd like.

INSTRUCTIONS

The following set of instructions is a blend of both the alcohol – which is conveyed in part one of the recipe – and the hot water as outlined in part two. This is the "ultimate" kind of tincture. It does require a bit of patience on your part in creating it – especially the first or second time you make it.

The other aspect to keep in mind is that this recipe is based on using a one-gallon of tincture, but this same recipe works any size jar. The key to success is to maintain the chaga to alcohol ratio balance. This is not a quick recipe, so that's why making a large batch at one time makes the most sense.

PART 1: ALCOHOL EXTRACTION

Take the chaga chunks and break them into roughly one-inch pieces. Grind these pieces into a powder, using a coffee or spice grinder, or if you'd like, a blender.

Place the ground chaga in a one-gallon glass jar, leaving approximately two inches of room. Now, fill this jar with vodka.

Allow this mixture to set for at least two months. But within this eight-week period, pay attention to it by shaking the jar every day.

PART 2 - HOT WATER EXTRACTION

Following the eight weeks of steeping, strain the alcohol from the glass jar into another glass jar. Using a cheesecloth is the perfect way to strain them.

Then take this alcohol-soaked chaga into a clay pot. You'll use the same amount of water that was strained in the previous step. Pour this water into a clay pot, then use a stick of some sort to measure the water level.

I use a chopstick and, using a knife, I carefully mark the water level on the eating utensil. This indicates the final water level you'll want to see once the tincture process is completed.

Now add water equal to what you already have into the pot. At this point, you should have double the amount of water you began with. Bring the pot to a boil. Then allow it to simmer on low heat.

Continue to check the water level using the chopstick you've marked. When the water level simmers down to what you had or even farther, you can take this off the stove and allow it to rest for 24 hours.

The following day, add yet more water and boil it down as you did before until you have less water than the day before. Repeat these steps for a total of three times. When the third decoction is complete, allow it to cool. Mix that with the alcohol you saved at the beginning of these instructions. You can store this in a glass jar.

Your tincture is now ready to use. You'll put one teaspoon of this tincture into eight ounces of liquid.

CHAPTER 6: CHAGA RECIPES

If you're interested in trying to get the healing nutrients and phytonutrients into your system as easily as possible, why not do what people have done for thousands of years, and drink it as a tea as often you would like?

With this habit in mind, I've included a few recipes that feature this mushroom.

CHAGA MUSHROOM TEA

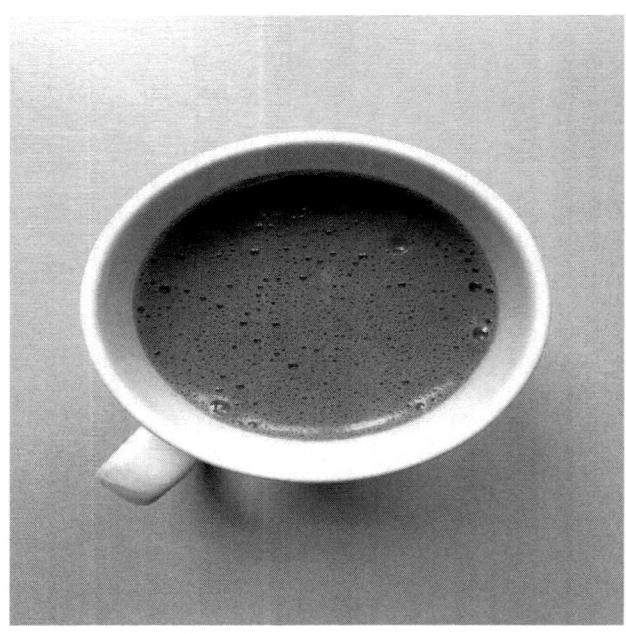

For this recipe, you'll want to use either the entire chunks of mushroom or you can grind them into a powder with your coffee grinder if you have one, or you can use two teaspoons of the powdered mushroom.

Single Serve

Until the Keurig Company makes a Chaga mushroom tea K-Cup for its coffee-making machine, you'll have to make the tea the old-fashioned way, by steeping its ingredients.

Place either a chunk of the chaga or the ground version into an empty mug.

Fill the cup with boiling water over the mushroom. Allow this to steep for at least three minutes. If you like your tea a bit stronger, then you may steep it a longer than this.

Add lemon, raw honey, or even natural maple syrup to taste.

This one is our favorite summer recipes. There are two types of people in the world – one type likes hot food and drink in summer, the other type doesn't.

We personally prefer **cool, cold drinks** on hot days. Hot drinks just make you sweat and raise your core body temperature, and perhaps lead to dehydration.

Ingredients:

1 teaspoon Chaga powder per cup of ice tea
Maple syrup, honey, lemon, to taste
Ice cube

Directions:

Make hot Chaga tea using the previous steps.
Add maple syrup or honey (or both) to taste.
Allow it to cool for 15-30 minutes.
Pour the tea in a container.

To cool, place this container in the freezer for no more than 45 minutes to an hour.

After this, add ice cubes and lemon.

Morning cup of Coffee a la Chaga

If you love your morning cup of Joe as much as I do (okay, I crave my morning coffee) you may not even glance at this recipe. After all, nothing can take the place of your first satisfying cup of coffee in the morning.

But you needn't worry about your coffee craving. It's a mixture of your favorite coffee with Chaga added. It's a veritable explosion of flavor, the flavors of the coffee blends to perfection with the earthy aroma and taste of the Chaga.

Ingredients:

Your favorite coffee (I prefer a full-bodied French roast, but it works with any blend of coffee)
1 teaspoon of chaga per cup of coffee

Directions:

Make your coffee as usual.

Add one teaspoon of chaga into the coffee maker per cup. If you are making six cups of coffee, for example, you'll add one teaspoon of the mushroom.

Allow this to simmer for a short time before you begin to enjoy it.

CHAGA CHAI TEA

Ingredients:
8 oz. of chai tea
2 teaspoons of Chaga powder
1 tablespoon of coconut and cinnamon
Sweeten to taste

Place all the ingredients on a blender and blend until the mixture is smooth.

You can enjoy this – like any other Chai tea – either hot or cold, depending on your mood.

LEMON CHAGA WATER

Some days, even on some of the hottest of days, all you really want to drink is an ice-cold glass of water.

Nutritionists tell us that water is the best way to keep us hydrated. So, why not? Lemon Chaga water. Here's how I prepare mine and it's proven to be my go-to drink when the weather gets unseasonably or unbearably hot.

Ingredients:

1 lemon

Ice cubes

Water

1 teaspoon Chaga extract

Using a pitcher or carafe, fill it three-quarters full with water.

Cut the lemon into wedges. Place half of these wedges into the pitcher. Squeeze the other half into the water. Add the ice cubes.

Add approximately 8 teaspoons of chaga tincture to the water.

CHUG-A-CHAGA SMOOTHIE

Love smoothies? You're not alone – smoothies are quickly becoming one of the most popular drinks in the United States. The industry itself is making $2 billion years. Who among us hasn't stopped while we were shopping or during a long car trip and refueled our bodies through one of these drinks?

The beauty of a chaga smoothie isn't just the fact that you can enjoy it whenever you want in the privacy of your home, but you have control over all the ingredients. You can be sure nothing but healthy and fresh ingredients are in it. And you can make it to your specific taste.
And now, of course, you can include chaga and make it even a healthier drink. Remember that just because it's called a chaga smoothie, that the mushroom needs to have the leading role. Even a small amount can help to improve the healing power of these potent drinks.

The recipe below includes bananas, mangos, and strawberries, but feel free to make a smoothie with your favorites. Then add the amount of chaga shown below.

Ingredients:

1 cup coconut milk

1 banana

1 mango

5 large strawberries

Chaga tincture

Directions:

Put all the ingredients (with the exception of the chaga) into a blender. If you normally add ice cubes, you can do that now.

Blend this until it's smooth.

Add 15 drops of chaga tincture and blend a bit more.

HONEY-CHAGA MUFFINS

What's your morning coffee or smoothie without a delicious muffin to go with it? There's something not quite right about this. So, that's why we're introducing you to a chaga muffin recipe. You may want to start off baking the one below, but as you get more familiar with these muffins, you'll be incorporating chaga into all of your favorite muffin recipes. And now there's no reason not to!

The recipe I suggest below normally makes approximately a dozen muffins and takes only about a half hour of your time. Now that's the start of a good morning!

Ingredients:

2 cups all-purpose flour

3 teaspoons baking powder

½ teaspoon salt

1 cup honey

1 egg

1 cup of milk

¼ cup vegetable oil

6 teaspoons of Chaga extract or tincture.

Preheat the oven to 400 degrees Fahrenheit.

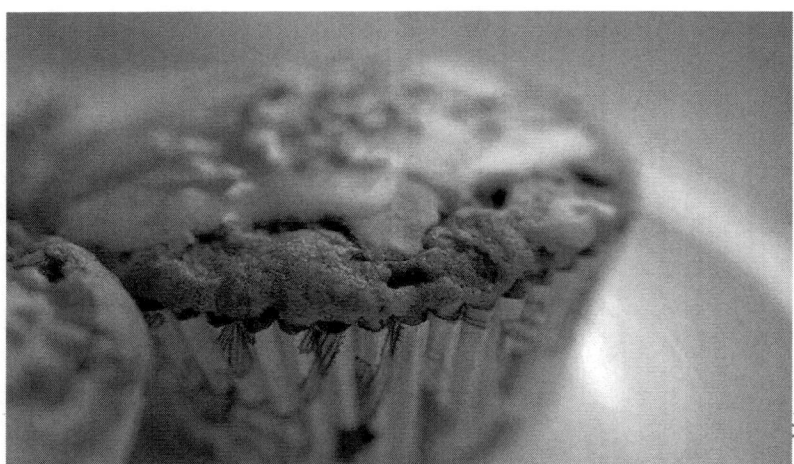

Place the following ingredients in a large mixing bowl: the flour, baking powder, salt, and sugar.

In another smaller mixing bowl, beat the egg with a fork, then stir the milk and oil into the egg.

Combine the liquid ingredients with the dry ones in the larger bowl. Add the Chaga..

Using a fork, fold all the ingredients together gently until the entire mixture is moistened.
Take this batter and pour it into a muffin pan that has already been lined with paper cups.

Bake these for 25 minutes or until the tops are golden brown.

"HEALTHY" CHOCOLATE ICE CREAM

You know you're going to eat it.

There's something undeniably decadent about ice cream. And admit it, whether it's good for you or not, you're going to have at the very least a couple of tastes of ice cream.

So why not make your own and make it as healthy as ice cream could be?

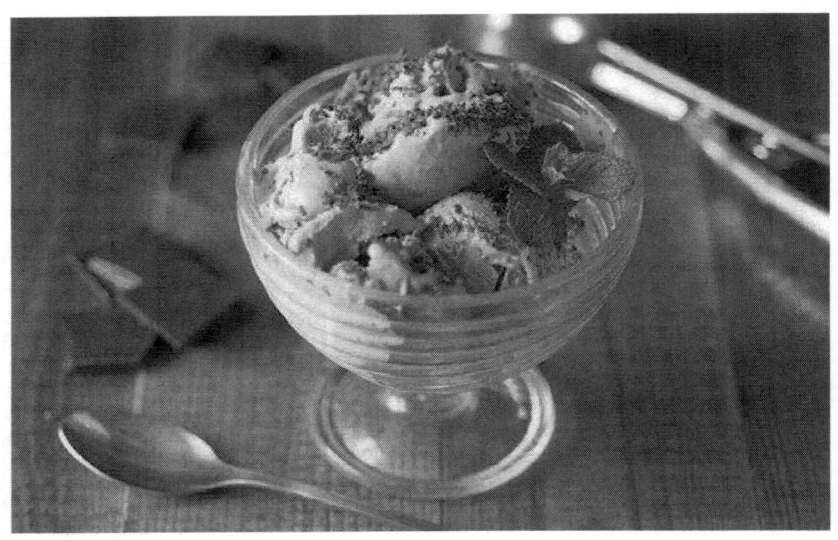

That includes not only organic when possible, but also the potent health-giving ingredients chaga has to offer. Don't think it's possible? Try the ice cream recipe below that is if you're not afraid of becoming a believer.

Ingredients:

3 bananas

4 oz. chocolate

1 cup heavy cream

1 teaspoon organic cocoa powder

2 tsp Chaga extract or tincture.

Directions:

Mix all the ingredients in a blender and blend until the texture is smooth.

If this doesn't result in a mixture that's sufficiently smooth, then add a bit of sugar and real cream, and pour the result into an ice cream maker.

RUM AND COLA WITH CHAGA

The following recipe should have a great big neon sign next to it. Why? Because it's an alcoholic based drink. It should not be consumed by children or young adults under your state's legal drinking age. And of course, if you're a recovering alcoholic who fears of slipping into another drinking cycle, then under no circumstances is this drink for you.

But if you have no inherent problem with alcoholic drinks, either physically, emotionally, or even religiously, then a rum and cola is the best place to start on making that relaxing drink do a bit of some healthy work through the addition of chaga.

Ingredients:

2 oz. Rum
Cola
1 Lime
Ice cubes
Chaga extract

Take half of the lime and squeeze the juice into the bottom of a glass.
Take the chaga extract or tincture and put it in the glass with the lemon juice.
Add the two ounces of rum.
Add the cola, to suit your taste. Then add ice cubes.

It's that easy to take a popular alcoholic drink and fortify it with chaga.

If you already drink rum and cola, you'll discover that this drink is to be consumed with care. For some reason, the alcohol in this drink may have a larger effect on your body than usual.

One more warning: if you're currently taking any prescription medication before you sip on this, ensure you're not causing your body any undue harm by taking a herb that has the potential to cause adverse side effects.

CONCLUSION

The mushroom of immortality. A gift from God. A diamond of the forest.

Whatever it's been called through history and in various cultures, there's not a doubt among the indigenous people that chaga is a very special fungus. In cultures that live long, healthy lives and whose ancestors have also enjoyed this type of life for thousands of years, there is a single thread that runs through their longevity. Their long lives are based on their use of herbal and natural medicine. Chaga is not considered "just another herb or mushroom." It's revered and honored for its health-giving qualities.

You don't have to know the language of these people, or their other natural remedies to recognize from these monikers that chaga stands in a class of its own.

We've seen, even in the short time we've had together in this book, how both anecdotal and now a growing amount of scientific studies are binding together to form a powerful argument for the one-of-a-kind healing herb that has helped individuals from tsars to peasants, from the secular to the spiritual – to not only maintain health but also improve it.

The bottom line here is that the unassuming but powerful fungus has seemingly eliminated symptoms and healed a diverse array of seemingly unrelated disorders.

For far too many years, generations even, the mushroom's qualities were either ignored or met with disbelief. When I faced the serious health challenge that is cancer, I decided to give this mushroom a try. When I got the nod from my oncologist, I began my healing routine each morning with chaga tea.

I worked my way up to 8 to 10 cups a day. After certain milestones in my treatment and the improvement in my health, I reduced this to a maintenance serving of no less than six cups daily, even seven years after the surgery and chemotherapy. Of course, I've added a host of other changes as well, but I believe I owe my health today to my daily meditation, positive affirmations, and my generous use of chaga. I've learned how to not only drink the tea but also how to add to any number of foods, from smoothies to main meals and desserts.

What I hope you take away from this book is that science is hustling to get caught up with the overwhelming anecdotal evidence, the word of mouth stories passed from generation to generation about this jewel of the forest, as well as nods of appreciation from novelists who chose to include remarks in their writings. These scientific studies are beginning to crack the code of the mushroom's legendary potency, isolating many of the enzymes, phytonutrients, and other essential substances for outstanding health.

If you were skeptical upon first learning about chaga, you were well within your bounds to be. It's hard to believe that any herb or food that has so many claims clamped on to it can be that beneficial in reality.

To be quite honest, it very well could be that you'll start using chaga only to discover it doesn't work on you as well as it does for others. After all, each of our bodies is unique and processes nutrients and other essential dietary needs differently. My bet, though, is on the chaga. At least one of its amazing healing characteristics will prove to be useful for improving your health or kick starting you into an unbelievable new level of well-being.

I like to think I'm living proof that chaga is still working wonders today.

Printed in Great Britain
by Amazon

31305988R00062